T.S.G., E.D.G. and ME

Our Journey Through Pregnancy and Postpartum Psychosis

by
Jennifer Goodman

Bloomington, IN  Milton Keynes, UK

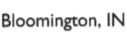
authorHOUSE™

AuthorHouse™
1663 Liberty Drive, Suite 200
Bloomington, IN 47403
www.authorhouse.com
Phone: 1-800-839-8640

AuthorHouse™ UK Ltd.
500 Avebury Boulevard
Central Milton Keynes, MK9 2BE
www.authorhouse.co.uk
Phone: 08001974150

First published by AuthorHouse 1/16/2007

ISBN: 978-1-4259-7790-0 (sc)

Printed in the United States of America
Bloomington, Indiana

This book is printed on acid-free paper.

My book has two dedications.

To mommy's miracle from God.

To my Grammy, you are not forgotten; you are forever in my heart always and forever. I love and miss you everyday.

The Thank Yous!!!!

Anyone that knows me knows I like to give credit where credit is due and thank people along the way.

I would have to thank God first because I felt so creative when I first knew I was pregnant. I have never felt so creative in my life. You really do work hand and hand from conception to delivery with God.

To my husband, you are my rock. Now I understand what true love is. You are the most unselfish person I know and hardworking. I will love you forever and always. Thank you for the support. I know it wasn't easy.

Dad and Mom, Thank you for the love that you have for me. I am and will always be your firstborn.

To my 4 sisters, I am blessed to have sisters like you. Thank you for putting up with all of my emotions. I love you all in different ways.

To my in-laws: Thank you for raising a fine young man. Thanks for the dinners on Monday nights Joyce☺ How thoughtful of you. I love you guys.

Kristen and Simon: We miss you! Enjoy Colorado.

There are many people who helped me and inspired me with this dream of mine to write a book. Thank you to all of you. You know who you are.

Charlotte and Erin: Thanks for letting me talk about the stress in my life and all the drama going on. You guys are the best. I love you.

Ahren Owen: He is my Author Service Representative. Thanks for making my dream became a reality.

Last but not least I want to express my gratitude to the staff at the hospital. They handled all of my needs as well as my newborn son's needs superbly. Troy,E.D.G. and I want to thank-you from the bottom of our hearts.

Introduction

Hello to all my readers. How are you? I am 30 years old and I live in New Hampshire with my husband Troy and our newborn son. We are first time parents as you know. I thought I'd start by telling you a little about myself. I have been married to a wonderful, caring and supportive man for a little over 4 years now. We have been dating 6 years this coming January. I love him for the man that he is. I love that he looked passed my skin and saw my soul and fell in love with that person. He is the hardest working 30 year old I know! He is mentioned all the time in the book obviously.

I have 4 sisters. We all get along very well. We do have our differences and bicker but what woman doesn't. We are all very close. You will see when you read the book. Anyone that knows our family knows just how tight a bond we have a sisters. Having a sister is the best but having 4 is a blessing.

I have truly loving parents. They would do anything for their children. My mom and dad had me and Christine at an early age with not much money. Now I understand how overwhelming it is having a child of your own, but somehow they managed and we all turned out wonderful if I do say so myself.

I love my in laws. They are so hospitable. My mother in law cooks dinner every Monday night. She is a very caring person as well. My father in law is so funny. We like to joke around with each other.

And last but not least I am blessed with a great circle of friends. I can count on a few of them for anything. That is what a friend is all about. One friend came from Massachusetts to visit me in the hospital and another called from California. I love these girls like they were my own sisters. I hope they know that. Other friends that lived local called and visited. That always makes you feel so good and warm inside.

My primary goal for writing this memoir/autobiography is to help woman with bipolar who become pregnant. 1 in every 1000 pregnant woman who have bipolar develop postpartum psychosis. You can look at the resource section to have the illness defined to you but basically you have psychotic episodes. That is what I had. I also had delusions and acted bizarre.

It is a pretty frightening feeling for you, your spouse, family and friends. But beware it is TREATABLE. I was back to my old self within 3 or 4 weeks with support, medicine and therapy.

I wrote in a journal when I found out I was pregnant so that will be the style I choose to write in. I have written in journals for about 13 years now. It is very therapeutic. Well I would love to share my story with whoever is interested. So on with my story.

Weeks 1-13
(The First Trimester)

JANUARY 24, 2006

It is official!!! Troy and I are going to have a baby. I am so excited. Joyce went to the doctor's office with me. We tried two of the same pregnancy tests and they were defective but always said we were pregnant the next morning so that is why I made an appointment today with my doctor to see if we were pregnant and we are. I am on cloud 9. I immediately tracked down my mom with Joyce to tell her. She had a tear in her eye. Troy was going to call during his lunch break so I made sure I got home by noon. He called and he was so excited as well. He told everyone at work and the ladies all gave him hugs. Troy came home with a half dozen roses and a snoopy stuffed animal for the baby. He said it reminded him of a snoopy he had when he was a child. Jack gave us a stuffed seal and bath fishy toys. We went out to dinner to celebrate at the Outback Steakhouse with my mom and dad.

Excerpt from my journal:

It's official! I am pregnant. Hurray. Thank you God and Grammy. I know you made this real and true. I love you. I will write later. I have to eat lunch now. Erin sent us an e-card, and wished us congratulations on the baby news. Joyce gave us a binkie and some spoons and bowls.

WEEK 5

We found out the due date. It is October 1,2006. Wednesday or Thursday (I saw a slight trace of blood). I have slight cramps on the bottom left side of my stomach. I cried when I talked to mom about my sisters not showing their excitement for our baby coming. Must be my hormones raging. My poor husband. Sorry troy. Dad and mom bought us a teddy bear that puts his hands together and says a prayer and lights up. It is musical (twinkle, twinkle little star). Charlotte and Kevin sent us a card. Erin sent an e-card to me.

WEEK 6

Sat. 2/4/06 I had slight cramps throughout the day and some slight signs of blood at around 4:30pm. Sunday, no cramps yet. Sunday 2/5/06 I felt a little nauseous. I think it was the chicken finger dinner. Wednesday 2/9/06 I didn't really like the smell of the bbq grill. Mickayla and Jeff sent us a card. Charlie and Joyce gave us a cabbage patch kid from 1985. They saved it for their first granddaughter. We will find out the sex during the 18th week.

WEEK 7

Our first ultrasound visit on 2/14/06 (Valentines Day). I saw the baby for the first and heard their heartbeat. It was incredible. My mom told dad I was glowing. People have told me that I am glowing. A coworker says hey sparkly to me when I see her. The pregnancy felt completely real after I saw the baby on the screen and heard their heartbeat. Grammy Joyce and Bumpa bought the baby a monitor for a Valentine's Day gift. Cool huh! We got the first ultrasound pictures.

Excerpt from my journal:

We had dinner with my dad at Buckey's. He is going to Myrtle Beach for awhile. Watch over him please. I love him tons. He likes the weather down there during the winter months.

WEEK 8

Tuesday I went to a fast food restaurant and threw up a little in the public bathroom. Yuck. We had problems with our drains at work on Friday, the smell was awful. I protected our baby as much as I could. I love being pregnant for the first time. I want to thank god for this miracle. Please let Troy and I raise a wonderful child together. Auntie Lynn and Uncle George won us a basket with safety first baby stuff in it. Cool huh?

WEEK 9

Gene and Maura gave us a bunch of baby stuff for our baby. We have such good friends. Cool huh? Nicole and Marybeth congratulated Troy and I. They said I was going to be a good mom. That means so much to me.

Week 11

Mommy got sick today at work. She took the trash from the ladies room out to the truck and went back to work as usual. Troy and I had our first argument while I was pregnant. This is not good for the baby, Troy, or I.

Excerpt from journal:

I love being pregnant. It is such a miracle. Thank you God for all of this. You made Troy and I very happy. We will be the best parents to our baby. God, say hello to Grammy please.

Week 12

During week 11, I made my sisters a special gift from the heart. I thought of it while I was pregnant. I feel so creative being pregnant. Troy noticed that I was beginning to show around this week. It is hard to tell because I am obese and all. He said my stomach felt more firm and hard to him. That is cool.

WEEK 13

There are a lot of women that I know who are pregnant this year or who were pregnant this year. The first trimester is over. Two more to go. Thank you for the little miracle growing inside of me. Goodnight God.

Excerpt from my journal:

Troy and I are still very happy about our pregnancy. . The first trimester is over. Two more to go. Thank you for the little miracle growing inside of me. Goodnight God. The first trimester went very well.

Weeks (14-26)
The Second
Trimester

WEEK 14

I heard your heartbeat today. We can find out if you are a boy or a girl on Wednesday may 3, 2006. Daddy and I are very excited little one. Happy 21st Aunt Shawna!!! I was the designated driver for Shawna's 21st birthday party. We went to Portland. Aunt Lynn was the other designated driver. We had a good time. It was a late night though. You heard the loud music inside my belly. The bars are smoke free in Portland. I would not have gone if they were not.

Week 15

Grandma and mommy went to NYC to see the Phantom of the Opera on Broadway. It was spectacular. I think you enjoyed the music. We bonded all the way down. I love your grandmother so much. She knows that. As far as the subways and buses go God was on our side. We made it to our hotel with just enough time to get ready and head into the city. The show was phenomenal. The music is soulful and breathtaking. Grandma is the best. We were supposed to go on a harbor cruise to see the Statue of Liberty but it rained that day so we headed home. We had dinner at a Japanese restaurant. It was very entertaining. Mom had them bring out a slice of cheesecake and have them wish me a happy birthday. Then I thought I was going to Aunt Shawna and uncle Jeff's for a bbq. It was a surprise 30th birthday for me. My family was there except for dad because he was in Myrtle Beach. Some friends were there. I was so shocked and happy.

Week 16 and 17

The doctor's office called and said my glucose (blood sugar) level was high. I have to eat normal for the next 3 days but I have to eat 2 candy bars each day. Then I go in on the third day and have my blood drawn 4 times. Troy got all nervous when he heard this. Oh daddy bought mommy this beautiful tanzanite necklace she wanted for her birthday. Daddy spoils mommy. We went to visit Charlotte's condo in Medford and ate at the Tavern On the Water. We had iced coffees at Starbucks and went into a shop called Urban Trends. Mommy had fun with her friend. She has known her for 25 years. Wow!!!

WEEK 18

And the sex is??? You are a boy. Daddy said yes in the doctor's office. He was very excited. So was mommy. We told everyone. Before mommy had a chance to tell her sisters grandma already did. Mommy got upset a little but knows grandma is just excited and is a proud grandmother already.

Week 19

Daddy bought you a Dale Earnhardt Jr. #8 outfit. We bought your baby book too! Mommy bought you your first pair of Nike sneakers with the gift certificate Aunt Rachel gave mommy for her birthday.   Aunt Lynn and Mary gave me mother to be cards for Mother's day. Cute, huh? On 5/19/06 aunt Shawna graduated from NHTI. I bought you a bib in the book store. We are so proud of Aunt Shawna.

WEEK 20

Daddy and I can't wait to meet you. We love you so much already. We are going to be the happiest parents when we meet you. Stay healthy inside of mommy. Mommy's body isn't in good shape but I am sure you are fine inside of me. I am proud to be a part of this miraculous experience. Daddy is so happy too. Aunt Catherine talked to you and was touching mommy's belly. It was a nice moment. She said Uncle Jeremy and her are going to buy you your first Red Sox outfit!

WEEK 21

One of mommy's best friends is pregnant. She is due December 10th. We have known each other since high school. We went bowling at Funspot with some of our friends. Troy's bowling ball fell out of his hand and hit the two poles. It bounced in between them and made a noise. It was hilarious. The people laughed. It was something. Troy and I celebrated our 4th wedding anniversary. He brought home some flowers and we went out to dinner. Then we played mini golf. It was a lot of fun.

WEEK 22

Aunt Shawna, Aunt Lynn and mommy went to the drive-in at the Weirs to see the Da Vinci code. We had a lot of fun. Aunt Shawna and mommy saw Martina McBride at Meadow Brook in Gilford, NH. You were moving and kicking a lot during that concert. You enjoyed the concert just like your mom and aunt did. Aunt Shawna rubbed the 50/50 ticket on mommy's belly for good luck but she didn't win.

Excerpt from my journal:

On June 4, 2006 I felt you move for the first time. You probably moved before this day but this is when I first remember the feeling. I was lying in bed because it was my day off from work and I just felt you kick. It was miraculous. I could not wait to tell your daddy. What a gift from God. Thanks for that experience God.

WEEK 23

Daddy is going to NYC with Evan on Saturday 6/10/2006. He is seeing One Night Stand. It is a wrestling show. He will take you when you get older. He is so excited. On Tuesday June 4,2006 that is when I felt you move for the first time. Daddy called from NYC and had me put the answering machine to my belly so you could hear his voice. Cool huh?

Week 24

Not too much happened this week!!!!

WEEK 25

Daddy received his first father to be card from mommy. He liked that. We went to Grammy Joyce and Bumpa's on Monday night to drop off a Father's Day card and celebrate Father's Day. We had bbq the day before at grandma and grandpa's house. We had fun at both places.

Excerpt from my journal:

Grandma quit her job. She was there 11 years. She is on her way to Myrtle Beach with Aunt Lynn. She is kind of going through something right now. Please be with her God and guide her. We all love her so much.

WEEK 26

Mommy's friend Jen gave us a car seat and a whole bunch of other stuff for you. She is very nice and it was very thoughtful of her and her family. There have been so many generous people out there who love and care about us. We are truly blessed.

Weeks (27-37)
The Third Trimester

Also titled
(When All Hell Broke Loose JK)

Week 27

Daddy and I ate dinner at Friendly's. We had a nice time. Then we went to Wal-Mart.

Week 28

You keep moving around a lot. It is so miraculous. I love the feeling. Mommy will cough and sometimes she pees a little. How embarrassing. Women go through so much don't they??? Daddy asked me if you kicked or were moving and I said not really then all of a sudden you moved. It was like you heard us talking or something. It was so cool. You are moving a lot now!!!

Week 29

Today mommy found out that her blood sugar test came back positive. The doctors told her she has gestational diabetes. She just wants support from her friends and family. She thought this might happen.

Excerpt from my journal:

I have had a wonderful pregnancy so far. I am 30 weeks pregnant so far. Last Friday I caught a cold from one of the two guys I work with and I can't smell anything or really taste the food I enjoy eating. It has been over a week now. E.D.G. (our baby boy) is moving a lot lately. We love him so much. We can't wait to see him for the first time. I love being pregnant. Thank you for creating a life with Troy and I. We will be the best parents to our baby boy. I promise you that god. God bless everyone that I love and care about.

Week 30

Friday July 28, 2006 was when I started to feel a pain near my rib cage. It is one of your body parts I guess. That was Aunt Catherine's 29th Birthday.

Week 31

We had another ultrasound on Wednesday august 2nd (Bumpa's Birthday). You are around 4 lbs or so. I have high blood pressure so the doctor told me to take a few days off from work. Aunt Liz is here. She is doing chores for mommy because the doctors want me to rest. Oh daddy, Aunt Shawna, Aunt lynn, Grandma and mommy saw you on the ultrasound machine. It was special time for all of us.

Excerpt from my journal:

7/31/06

Troy is going to quit his job. He hasn't been happy there so he is going to type a letter of resignation and give it to the human resources department tomorrow. I am proud of him. He works too hard. He should love what he does. Please watch over him God. He would have been there 7 years this coming November.

Week 32

8/2/06

Today was Bumpa's birthday. Simon is home visiting from Colorado. He gets bigger and bigger every year. He is such a good boy.

8/5/06

Mommy called daddy at aunt Shawna's and uncle jeff's house cause he was playing cards there. It was 11 pm and he wasn't home yet. Your foot was STILL hurting my side and back so I was upset with daddy for not being around when I wanted him. HORMONES again. On 8/5/06 the doctors put me on Labetalol to lower my blood pressure.

8/6/06

On Sunday daddy felt you move. You are a very active boy.

8/10/06

Today was our baby shower. My hormones went crazy that night? The ladies did a wonderful job. Everything was perfect. We received so many beautiful gifts. Thanks to everyone who made things and bought things to make the day special to troy, the baby and I. We truly are grateful.

Mommy was relaxing at the Melvin Wharf when she met a lady walking her 5 week old with her mother. It doesn't get anymore relaxing than that huh?

WEEK 33

It is Grammy Joyce's birthday today. We had lobsters with aunt Kristen because she is home for a week. We miss her a lot. Your cousin Simon is home too but he comes home for 4 weeks or so. You will meet him next time he comes home. He is going to love you!!!

8/7/06

Aunt Lynn came over and brought over her fan. It was very hot and humid in our house. She brought over Tylenol too for my rib that was still hurting from the way you were positioned. She bought dinner food and made it. She is an angel. What an unselfish girl huh? She also cleaned my whole house because the doctor didn't want me to do anything major. They just want me to put my feet up. Aunt Rachel brought me a shake over from Ben and Jerry's. Thanks Aunt Rachel. You are the best.

8/16/06

I cried in the doctors office with Troy and the doctor. I am a little stressed because they want me to relax. I don't really know how to relax. I have always been on the go but Troy's family is more low key than my family. They know how to relax. The doctors don't want me to do too much. I have to collect my urine for 24 hours again and then I go to bring it to the lab on Friday morning. Hang on little buddy. I will meet you very soon. Uncle George is 21 today. They came over last night for dinner and cake. Daddy and the boys played Texas Hold'em.

8/13/06

We went to a bbq at Uncle Jeff and Aunt Shawna's house. We had a nice time.

Daddy quit his job. He worked there almost 7 years. Mommy is so proud of daddy. She wants daddy to be happy and he wasn't happy there towards the end. She tried to get some of his work buddies and friends together but it didn't work out. She sent him flowers to work. He got embarrassed I am sure.

WEEK 34

On 8/19/06 daddy started to work on your nursery. We bought a Snoopy border for the walls and that is the theme we chose for your room. He is doing a wonderful job. We love him so much huh?

On 8/23/06 Grammy Joyce and daddy were at your 4th ultrasound. How exciting. You are probably around 5 lbs 10 ounces he said. We can't wait until you are born.

Week 35

Aunt Shawna had her bridal shower at the club. Aunt Catherine made two beautiful cakes. She made two pretty cakes for our baby shower. Aunt Catherine and Aunt Lynn really did a wonderful job making Shawna's shower a success. There were other people who helped with preparing for Aunt Shawna's bridal shower but Aunt Catherine and Aunt Lynn did most the work. The shower was a lot of fun. Aunt Shawna enjoyed herself.

Excerpt from my journal

8/18/06

Daddy bought all the groceries today and put the bags in and out of the car and put all the groceries away. He is our hero. The doctors tell me to just RELAX.

WEEK 36

We found out today with all the tests we did that that I got pre-eclampsia. The doctor said we will be induced next Tuesday 9/12/06. Yay. There is a light at the end of the tunnel. We are going to meet you soon. We are very excited. You have a nickname from one of the nurses because they have a hard time finding your heart rate on the fetal monitor. She calls you hidden Glidden. Cute, huh. Grandpa and grandma bought your crib on 9/7/06. It is beautiful. Your nursery is almost finished. There are a few things we can do later.

WEEK 37

Daddy and I ate at Louis Pizza before going to the hospital on Tuesday 9/12/06. We were excited because we were finally going to meet our unborn son. We arrived at the hospital at around 5:30pm or so. We got all settled in and the nurses we so hospitable. I really don't remember too much so bear with me. The doctor had to put a fetal electrode on our baby's head to measure his heart rate. I was already dilated 1 ½-2 cm so they gave me pitocin to start the induction. After that I just waited and listened to some relaxing music.

My husband and sister Lynn were with me but they went and chilled out in another room. They came in to see me a lot but not much was going to happen for a bit I guess.

By 9 am weds. Morning I was 7 or 8 cm dilated I think. It was getting time to push. I received an epidural. I loved that drug. I could not feel the contractions at all. The doctors came in and I told them I needed to push. I pushed for 30 minutes or so I don't know. Like I said I don't remember. Our son was stuck near my pelvic bone so we ended up having a caesarean section.

They had to knock me out for that because I could feel the pain a little. I remember talking to the anesthesiologist. I remember seeing the big light above me and then I just remember being in the recovery room. Everyone had seen our son before me because I had to go to the recovery room.

I remember being wheeled back into the maternity ward into my room. Troy was out smoking a cigarette. They wheeled E. D.G. into my room and I held him for the first time and then looked over at my sister Christine who had tears in her eyes which made me have tears in my eyes. They had to draw blood from him because they were checking his blood sugar. It came back fine. Thank God. I was on so many drugs I could not fully enjoy my brand new baby nor did I know what I was in store for next. My dad was checking my lower legs to see if the swelling was going down because I ended up getting pre-eclampsia like I said earlier.

A lot of friends and family members came to visit us and a lot of people brought us stuff. We had a lot of people who were concerned about us. Mommy doesn't remember a lot because she was on morphine the first 2 days and a lot of other drugs the rest of the days.

Postpartum psychosis
what??????

There are a lot of things in the hospital that I don't remember. From what I understand that is normal with all that I went through physically, emotionally and mentally. I personally think I started to lose it when I needed assistance from the nurses to help me breastfeed E.D.G. My brain chemistry acts different when I am under extreme stress. There was other stress in my life but I am not going to discuss that. Let's see we went into the hospital Tuesday l 9/12/06 and by Friday 9/15/06 that is when all the things started to unravel. I did call my doctor to let him know I thought I was going to need meds. I thought maybe I was getting postpartum depression because I have bipolar and they say you are at a greater risk of getting this illness. He spoke with my primary care physician and they started to put me on meds. I told my mom and Troy and they wanted me to rest that day. I took the day off from the baby I think and visitors too. My dad visited me and that is when things got weird. I became withdrawn from the baby. Then delusions started to happen and I was psychotic I guess. I thought my dad was my husband. I asked him if he was my husband. He said no. My Grammy passed away on December 8, 2004 mind you. And I guess I told a family member I was taking the baby to see her in Massachusetts. I thought I was my grandmother. My mother and Troy told me I spit out roast beef and said I just died. Later in the evening I peed the hospital bed and when the nurse and my father left the room I went to break the light or light bulb above the sink in my hospital room. I thought I saw the light and god was calling me home. Weird huh? Yeah I am still trying to grasp it but my therapist and friend says don't dwell on it. So I try not to but it is so bizarre. The brain is a powerful thing. My husband did not know what was going on. He had to leave and talk to friends and family I guess? My mother stayed in the room next door to me. During my whole psychotic phase they gave me a drug to have me come back to reality. I woke up that Saturday morning at around 1 am or so and saw a nurse outside my room with E.D.G. I was back to myself. Naturally I asked questions and my mom kind of filled in the blanks for me again. I just wanted to see my baby because I felt like I missed a lot of time with him. Troy came back to the hospital at 7 am. I just looked into his blue/green eyes and saw how scared and worried he really was. That is true love when you sense how your husband is feeling when you aren't feeling your best. It is also true love when the same man stays by your side in sickness and in health. I love you Troy. He is my rock. I think I took another shower on Saturday and that just felt awesome. The doctors came in and asked me questions. They asked if I wanted to harm myself or the baby. They have to ask you all these questions. I said no to both questions. They told me what had happened Friday night. I did not really know what postpartum psychosis was. One doctor found information online about this condition and printed it for me. On Sunday I got some more news. My doctor said I was anemic and I needed blood. I lost some blood during the c-section. I was supposed to be discharged on Monday 9/17/06. She was saying I might have to stay if I didn't have a blood transfusion and I started to cry. I received the blood on Sunday. They gave me 2 units. We finally left the hospital at 8pm or so on Monday 9/17/06. I was so happy. I was too cooped up. The service was phenomenal though.

Afterword

Our baby is 4 weeks old on Wednesday 10/18/06. He truly is a gift from God. I can't describe the experience of becoming a mother. I love him more and more each day. I can gaze in his eyes forever. He is always doing cool things and will constantly change. The first few weeks of pregnancy I knew something miraculous was happening. Anyways I can go on and on about motherhood.

Like I said in the beginning if you think you are experiencing any symptoms of postpartum depression or postpartum psychosis then seek help immediately. It is out there. There is a LIGHT at the end of the tunnel and other women are or have experienced this. This goes for all the dads out there too. Women need and love your support. Step up to the plate! Right hun??? You are not ALONE!!! I can't stress this enough and it is normal.

Postpartum Depression is more common than Postpartum Psychosis. Both are very treatable but I can't stress that you seek help IMMEDIATELY!!!

Resources:

BOOKS:

Down came the rain (my journey through postpartum depression) Brooke Shields

Beth: (A story of postpartum psychosis) Shirley Cervene Halvorson

The mother of all pregnancy organizers (Ann Douglas)

Your pregnancy week by week (dr. glade b. Curtis, ob/gy and Judith Schuler, ms

WEBSITES:

Postpartum.net

Bipolarhelpcenter.com

Pregnancy-info.net

Peaceandhealing.com

Charityadvantage.com

Melaniesbattle.org

Healthyplace.com

HOTLINES:

1-800-SUICIDE
1-800-7842433

1-800-PPD-MOMS
1-800-773-6667

1-800-273-TALK
1-800-273-8255

1-800-944-4PPD
1-800-944-4773

POSTPARTUM STRESS CENTER
1-610-525-7527

DEPRESSION AFTER DELIVERY(D.A.D.)
1-800-944-4773

POSTPARTUM SUPPORT INTERNATIONAL
1-805-967-7636

NATIONAL INSTITUTE OF MENTAL HEALTH
1-800-421-4211